time I released this book. Soon my team and I will be refining the first book I wrote and republish it. However, I know many of you want to know a lot about my surgery, the testing journey, recovery, seizure activity, and all the related things so my focus is getting the series out for you to know all the details at your own pace on your own schedule. I am not a professional in any field related to epilepsy but I have been declared one of the worst 30 cases in the United States since 2019. Turn the page to start reading my testimony based on my personal experience and journey.

Chapter 1

August 10, 2021

    In February 2020, I told my neurologist that I was tired of having seizures. I later found out she was an epileptologist, which is a neurologist that specializes only in epilepsy. I told her that all epileptic medications on the market had failed since my original diagnosis in October 1985. I had tried working with many doctors at different points throughout having my seizures or mental illnesses. These just worsened with all the different medications I tried having the Vagal Nerve Stimulator implanted six times. I was beyond tired of having seizures. I told my epileptologist that I would do whatever it took to no longer have epilepsy.

She warned my parents that this would be a ten month process of testings and that it would be years after surgery before "work and school could return to normal." On February 24, 2020 I was admitted to the Epilepsy Monitoring Unit of The Medical Center in Houston, Texas.

Upon admission to the hospital and arriving in the Epilepsy Monitoring Unit, the technician began gluing wires to my head, not allowing any hair products or hair pieces. I had to wear a button up or zip up shirt with my outfits and I was not allowed to get out of my bed without a registered nurse being in my room to attend, in case I were to have a seizure. He or she had to be with me to even watch me wipe myself down, since I was not allowed to take a bath or shower. The registered nurse had to also be in my room to attend while I went to the restroom, brushed my teeth and any other reason that I had to get out of bed. He or she had to be in the room for me to do anything and everything basically. I had zero independence.

At the same time as having to give up my independence, being in an unfamiliar environment, and so many other things being different about this situation, I was having my autistic episodes because my autism was causing an inability to deal with change or being off my regular routine. At the time, I also struggled with communication due to my autism. Clearly I am a high-functioning autistic, but combining that with being one of the top 30 worst cases of epilepsy in 2020,

my Post Traumatic Stress Disorder
(PTSD), Generalized Anxiety Disorder,
and Paranoia, I had more than my share
of struggles in order to function.

At the same time not being
content with being bedridden and having
autistic episodes, the epileptologist
doctor stopped my epilepsy medication,
but I continued to take my mental
health, Irritable Bowel Syndrome,
hypothyroid, and all other medications
my other doctors had prescribed. The
doctor, multiple researchers, plus
residents came to my room everyday
trying to get "the good news of" me
"having a seizure so that we can collect
our data."

I felt like the only joys in this
situation were eating, writing my books,
and reading other authors' books. I am
not the type who is interested in videos,
television, movies or other popular

entertainment that's available in hospitals. Therefore, I did not feel like I had much to do with my lengthy time in the Epilepsy Monitoring Unit. This made it very hard missing a total of ten days of work and a couple weekends when I would usually being doing something fun.

As a business owner, I was worried about my staff needing me, or one of my tasks that I could not perform being needed by the team or a client. I was worried about my tutoring clients going to other tutors or tutoring companies instead of waiting for my return.

Chapter 2

Well, it was more than a fear! I ended up in the Epilepsy Monitoring Unit for ten days before I had a seizure and they collected the data needed to move me to the next step in the testing process. While I was in the hospital, the pandemic of 2020 hit and life has never been the same since then. With my autism and the lockdown in Texas already happening when I was released, I could not see my friends, get coffee, tutor my clients, etc. This major, sudden change that was taking affect on multiple areas of my life, and was so sudden, caused an extreme reaction of attempting suicide. After my release from the hospital on day two, I ran to my neighbor's house panicking while telling her I just attempted suicide. She immediately noticed my backpack and asked where I was going? I carry all of my material to write and tutor each day. I told her that I was going to Starbucks. She asked me which Starbucks I was headed to, and I told her, openly and honestly. Shianne, asked me for the address, which I gave her, and if anyone will be there with me? I told her, "Yes. Mr. Lawrence is on his way now. He said he is going to stay with me the whole time until I find the help I need. Then, he will help me get there by giving me a ride."

Next, I headed to that Starbucks finding Mr. Lawrence ready at a table with his coffee in his hand and a smile on his face ready to see me. He gave me a hug and walked with me through the line to get my coffee. We went to the

table where he left his coffee. I got my
computer out to start researching mental
health hospitals for at least an hour
before two Fort Bend County deputies
came in and asked the workers "Is
there anyone here by the name of
'Jenn?'" I went to this one Starbucks
almost everyday so the Starbucks'
employees were able to point me out.
After a short conversation with the
deputies, going over what I already
shared with you, the deputy took me to
the closest medical hospital for them to
first run tests to check my liver after I
had overdosed on two pain killers,
taking twice the amount that my
research said was lethal. The medical
doctors there explained that they had to
first bring me to the medical hospital
emergency room to test my liver
because that excessive dose I took of

both ibuprofen and naproxen sodium can cause liver damage.

Well, it turned out my liver was as healthy as a horse so another ambulance took me to the nearest mental hospital that took both of my medical insurances and had an available bed.

After spending about two weeks in the mental hospital, on March 17, 2020, I was released. It was in March that I was approved for Disability Income and began receiving benefits that April. I went back to move to the next step in my surgery testing process to eliminate the seizures. With the pandemic here, and the whole thing new, it was at least May of 2020 before we could make any progress on the testings for me to be considered for any kind of surgery.

Chapter 3

    In the summer of 2020, which I do not remember the exact order, I had a Magnetic Resonance Imaging (MRI) test, an outpatient Electroencephalogram (EEG) and a neuropsychological evaluation where I had to assemble different blocks to copy patterns. In the neuropsychological exam, I also had to put odd shaped sticks into a board with one hand at a time, testing each hand one at a time. I then had to draw shapes inside of squares on a paper with different shapes representing different letters of the alphabet to make a code. On this part of the assessment, I had to race the clock and the doctor's assistant actually started a stopwatch and then told me when to stop.

The neuropsychologist required his assistant to read different elementary words asking me to remember as many of them as I could. This was followed by repeating the vocabulary words that I had remembered back to him in any order upon him stopping reading the words to me. I remembered him testing my vocabulary by showing me images and I had to tell him what they were called. I remembered that in 2020, I did not know the word "harp", but I do now after my surgery. I remembered at some point, he pointed to different dots on this sheet of paper that had dots in different spots within each square on the piece of paper. There were ten squares with each square having six dots each in random places within the square. I had to point to the black circle where he did. I was not able to copy him the first time around. He would tell me which ones I got right and which ones I got wrong, and he told me which black circles were correct. Then I had to try to make corrections for the wrong ones. As it turned out I would also get wrong some of the ones that I had already gotten right to this point. We did this, with him pointing to the right ones, and asking me to copy again, at least three to five times before moving to the next test.

By now, the guy testing me moved to the next part of the test, then came back to ask me to point to the correct dot in the squares to the best of my memory. I do not know my exact results, but I still got some of the dots wrong. I felt like waiting caused me to forget more while I did not know his actual findings.

Chapter 4

August 26, 2021

On another part of the neuropsychological exam, I had to cross out certain letters on a sheet with probably hundreds of small letters mixed in random order with random distance between them. The person giving me the exam only allowed somewhere around thirty seconds to a minute to find, and cross out all of the certain letters on the sheet that I could find. I did not know how I scored on this originally, but I remember being overwhelmed and feeling more anxious than running my business or tutoring a student. I was intimidated by it, clearly.

There was a total of five hours of testing in the neuropsychological exam. That included taking a number of ten minute breaks being how overwhelmed I got with the exam and a twenty minute break to have lunch. I had a good size, larger than normal, breakfast that day to be ready for loads of brain work. It did not seem like my large breakfast was enough. I ate during every break, not just lunch break. My parents had to push me each time I took a break to go back to the test because of being exhausted, stressed, and overwhelmed the testing had made me mentally.

If you or a loved one has to get this done, be sure to take plenty of extra food and drinks for the whole family. It's nearly an all day appointment. I remember my appointment was set for 8:00 a.m. but we did not finish and get to leave until 3:00 p.m. that day.

Chapter 5

After this testing was over and done with, we went the next week to get a Positron emission tomography (PET) scan. I had to stay up late, like I did for the EEG, but this time, I had to remain awake. I do not recall whether they injected it or I had to drink a fluid, but there had to be this fluid that went to my brain causing my brain to show in different colors on the big equipment circling around my head, similar to the CAT scan or MRI scan. I had to lay as still as I could. I was not allowed to move anymore than what I had to in order to breathe.

My understanding is that the fluid caused my brain, via the scan, to show in different colors that resembled different activities going on in my brain. If I had not consumed the liquid, the image in the results would appear black and white like a typical CAT scan or MRI scan results. I remember I had to be in a much smaller room by myself for the PET scan compared to that of an MRI or CAT scan room. While laying still in this very uncomfortable flat place, the machine was going around at a fast pace, much like a CAT scan or MRI scan does. Similarly to getting a CAT scan or MRI scan, the technician would tell me when she was about to take images again, and when it stopped for a short while so I could get adjusted, and get some short relief. This exam was much like the CAT or MRI experience, if you are familiar with them. The main difference is the extra small room, and having to take in some type of liquid so the brain would show results in colors.

Because of my Generalized Anxiety Disorder and Asperger's, I was beyond anxious in the PET scan where I could not have family nearby or was not allowed to take my anxiety medication that my psychiatrist had me take as needed. I definitely needed it though! I was in need of my Atarax without being allowed to take it or do any of my coping methods like reading my books, listening to music, meeting up with my friends, and so forth. If you or your loved one has Generalized Anxiety Disorder or Asperger's, please talk to the person ahead of time telling him/her things about ways to cope using the mind or imagination. For example, picturing somewhere pleasant; singing favorite songs in your head; watching a favorite TV show replay in your mind; and other ways you come up with to help him/her cope. I was not aware of these things so the PET scan ended up being one of my most difficult and uncomfortable tests.

Chapter 6

     I have had MRI's, blood work, and EEG's done pretty much my entire life since I had epilepsy at ten months old. That said, I am used to them, as well as CAT scans. Being used to these procedures, I know what to expect and do not get as anxious when I get them done as when I had to get an unfamiliar exam done, and especially the PET scan where I was alone. I could not have anyone, anything, or any of my medications in that very small room 100% alone, unable to sit up, or move at all without the technicians having to scan again. My movements would mess up the images that the technicians were taking with the PET scan, even with the most minute motion or movement. As I remembered, I battled with the desire to die due to my Post Traumatic Stress Disorder (PTSD) and prior bad experiences like doctors wanting to kill me, and past rape and sexual assault experiences.

I also had paranoia that heightened my traumas making me think that the PET scan was the doctors' way of trying to kill me. I compared it, in my head, with the electric chairs criminals sit in when they get the death penalty. You may think that this is mostly because of my various mental illnesses. Research has shown a common link between epilepsy and mental illnesses. Researchers have also shown a link between autism and epilepsy, so I know my case of having more than one or all three of these types of conditions is not uncommon among epileptics.

Think about how each of the three types of conditions have to do with the brain not working correctly or completely. To me, that made sense. Either the brain does or does not work properly or fully. It does vary by the specific person; but I want you to understand why I insist on you helping prepare your loved one or yourself, for these various steps in getting ready for brain surgery.

In September 2020, I filed for Supplemental Nutritional Assistance Program (SNAP) which was approved. I received this program through a much easier and quicker process than most people. Some people still refer to SNAP as "Food Stamps" which was the former term. By October 2020, I had my SNAP debit card along with my first deposit and I bought some groceries. I had to admit it was not enough to eat three meals a day, but for sure bought more food than I could get on my Disability and Supplemental Security Income checks alone, even with the little bit I made working.

Chapter 7

   Another test I had was the Wada test. *Johns Hopkins definition is, "the Wada test can help a physician evaluate how important each side of the brain is with respect to language and memory functions. Data from the Wada test help the epilepsy team determine the approach most likely to address seizures while preserving areas of the brain associated with speech and memory."*

   For this test, I had to go to the hospital, throw on a hospital gown, and lay down on a hard surface with at least a dozen people around me in an operating room. Before starting the operation I was given an injection through a tube in the right half of my

groin area to make it numb. With the
area being numb, the injections he did
so many different times were not painful.
Next, there was an anesthesiologist who
injected fluid into my brain to sleep. I
only experienced discomfort when lying
down flat on the operating table; looking
downward to see a screen reading or
showing what I believed was my brain in
some kinds of images while other
images showing the inside areas of
where my injections were.

 After the sedation, I was not
anxious during this exam, even though
only one part of my brain was asleep,
because the sedation medication
relaxed me after it was injected and took
effect. One person who was at this
exam was visible to me at the command
of the anesthesiologist and my
neuropsychologist. There were other
people around I could see going in and

out of sight while I had no idea what role
they played or who they were. I had no
idea what role these other people
played in administering my Wada test.

   As far as the exam went, I
recalled feeling tired when he injected
the chemical and I naturally closed my
eyes thinking I was going to sleep, like
most of us at bedtime. Only within
seconds, my neuropsychologist said,
"Hey, Jenn. Are you still with us?" I
opened my eyes when I heard him ask
and made eye contact with him just to
my left. I responded with something
along the lines of "Yes?" or "I'm awake."
Next, my neuropsychologist gave me
directions to point to or read various
cards and I had to keep my focus on the
cards in his hand, doing just what he
directed. My neuropsychologist would
tell me what part of my brain had been
put to sleep each time there was

another injection. When the left side of my brain went to sleep, I could not move my limbs, talk, moan or anything. I could only look at the doctor making eye contact, unable to do anything more. I then heard one of the others in the operating room tell another person to mark the results on the exam "that the left half of the brain is dominant."

My neuropsychologist then said, "Okay, let's try putting only the front left temporal lobe to sleep." The anesthesiologist then gave me another injection. I woke and my neuropsychologist asked me again, "Jenn, are you with us?" I responded with something along the line of "Yes, I'm here." He then told me to read certain cards to him, which I did like the normal everyday me, and pointed to the dots or other shapes as he directed successfully like any ordinary day for myself. He directed me to point to certain things on the cards, and then touch my nose, followed by repeating this process with pointing to something different and back to touching my nose. I cannot tell you how many rounds we had of this one but I did all he asked like it was my everyday ritual. Clearly, to myself, I was functioning at my everyday ability with my front left temporal lobe asleep.

When they put the right half of my brain to sleep, I completed reading all the cards and pointed to shapes with no struggle. This confirmed that the left side of my brain was dominant as I was functioning fine with the entire right half of my brain asleep. This is very important. It is what told my surgeon that I would be able to function without a certain part of the left side of my brain. By removing the entire left half of my

brain it would further debilitate me
beyond my current level of already
being disabled.

As an extravert, I kind of liked the
Wada exam where I talked to people,
was the center of attention, and what I
had to do was elementary reading
material. Even the pointing was using
elementary level images and colors. I
am not saying I would want to go
through it again. It was not fun like my
hobbies, hanging out with my friends or
other preferred ways of enjoying my
time and life.

When I had my Wada test, it was
already October 2020 with the pandemic
still here; the lockdown temporarily over
with; cases of COVID-19 still
sky-rocketing, only now I personally had
even more to handle.

Chapter 8

Now my dad was in the hospital in the Intensive Care Unit with liver cancer. He retained high levels of fluid and doctors could not drain him of the fluids quick enough with the rate that his body stored the excessive amounts. All of these happenings around the local Houston, Texas area, the United States of America and around the world occurred, while I personally had my dad about to die. All this happened and went wrong at the same time put me into even worse depression. It was worse than what I suffered my first day home from the hospital when I attempted suicide.

By that time I was used to some of the new things about the world because of the pandemic so I called my psychiatrist, who put me on an additional antipsychotic medication as I always had opposite reactions to mood stabilizer medications, although PTSD is usually treated with mood stabilizers. Of course, my adverse reactions to medication is what had gotten me to the point with being considered for such major and risky surgeries. Just like mood stabilizers worsened my fight and flight mode episodes in severity and frequency, so did anti seizure or antiepileptic medications worsen the severity and frequency of my epileptic seizures.

By now, October 2020, I had my second severe seizure that landed me in the emergency room. Before that it was July, when I had a severe seizure on the toilet upstairs at my parents house, where I lived, for safety reasons; I cannot live alone. The seizure started while I was on the toilet and next thing my parents knew, I went running down the stairs until I fell breaking my left ankle.

Due to my broken left ankle, being in physical therapy, unable to walk, having to do all my tutoring at home now, I made up my mind that I would do whatever it took to be seizure free. I finally hit a point in my life with epilepsy that I had had enough of it. I decided, as anxious, depressed and uncomfortable all these tests made me, it was worth facing for the next two to three months if it meant that I could have hope of a life free of epilepsy, free of waking up not knowing where I was or how I had gotten there.

Going back not too long ago, I never saw hopes of being free of seizures. I had spent my whole life accepting epilepsy as being a part of me though I never enjoyed it. My mother said that I missed every three days of school in elementary, having at least five seizures each of those days. She said that I would forget everything the teachers had taught me each time I had a seizure so my mom spent hours at home reteaching me the material I forgot due to each seizure. It's my mother's belief that if she had not done this, I never would have graduated high school; much less have my college and graduate school education, which landed me in the profession of my dreams. I did not know how to determine the accuracy of what my mom claimed, but I knew my epilepsy had been a family struggle and not just mine.

Now I was ready for whatever it required to have hopes of a life free of

seizures, noting that I previously had
surgery six times. My hopes only led to
disappointment in not freeing me of
seizures. The six prior surgeries were all
implants of the latest version of the
Vagal Nerve Stimulator with my whole
family hoping, each time, that the latest
was better than the last, at making me
seizure free. My whole family feared me
reaching this point, exactly where I was
now, being considered for the most risky
type of last hope treatment to control my
epilepsy. My whole family was in fear of
this brain surgery, even through this
journey in testing to see what options I
had, if any, along with fears that it would
not work and we would all be out of
hope of life being better for any of us as
a family. We were at the end of our rope.
We had family fears that this journey
would make my PTSD worse, and
making my Seasonal Affected

Depression (SAD) worsen with a high risk of becoming more suicidal than ever before. This was an entire roller coaster ride, the scariest one possible, for my whole family.

We were struggling to keep ourselves together emotionally, and struggling to stay on track with the ten months of testing I had to do. The process of the constant testings each week risked my parents' jobs as they had to take me to all these tests which caused them to miss a lot of work days. Thanks to the Family and Medical Leave Act (FMLA), both of my parents were able to get medical documentation at the start of this process back in January 2020 when I asked my epileptologist to put me down this road.

With my epileptologist providing the proper documents for both of my parents' employers, they still had their jobs, and were both getting promotions while we were on this journey together. I, on the other hand, had a harder than usual time getting and keeping clients. A big part of it was because of the pandemic; another being because I was missing so much work for my seizures in combination with many doctor appointments for various tests and follow-ups. If it were not for my parents making enough extra money and fun money in their lines of work, this would have caused my tutoring, writing and business consulting company to shut down. With the fear of a possible shut down of my tutoring company, I started Books and More by Jennifer A. Whitaker, where you can find all my books. Books and More launched my writing career which was my new focus. My parents took me through this tough journey and saved my company so I

could continue to write and do other
work I loved.

Chapter 9

As you can see, Fall 2020 was a very difficult time for me. However, my tests did not stop there. I do not remember any tests or doctors' appointments in early to mid-November 2020 that had to do with the process leading up to finding my options of being seizure free. I remembered seeing my therapist one or two times a week for her to help me deal with the constant and extreme anxiety, fight flight mode, and depression related to the fear of my dad dying and my upcoming hospitalization in November 2020. I was also struggling at that time with finding and maintaining work that generated income with the on-going pandemic and my business looking like it would fail. Of course, I saw my therapist to deal with the changes I struggled to live with and accept that they were due to the pandemic.

At one point in October 2020 I tried to go to a partial hospitalization program, but, my mom, being a registered psych nurse, said that those kinds of programs always made me worse because they were not meant for people with autism and other neurological conditions. Those programs were meant for those who were only mentally ill and/or had drug problems. I have since then, tried other mental health treatment facilities, for some odd reason, and my mom continues to be proven right so I just worked more intensely with my outpatient therapist and psychiatrist.

I still saw my psychiatrist in November 2 020 as she had me visiting every four weeks at that point, in addition to seeing my therapist two times a week for more intensive outpatient care.

I went into the hospital on November 24th, which was the Monday before Thanksgiving. This time I was back in the Epilepsy Monitoring Unit at the medical hospital. I had chosen this date because my parents would already be off work and not have to miss any more work days, for this test at least, to help keep their jobs secure.

When I got to this hospital, I had to check-in, of course it included the COVID-19 questions, insurance information, billing information, and other paperwork. After all the regular stuff was done, the technician walked me back to the Epilepsy Monitoring Unit, and into my room. By now, I had been to the Memorial Hermann Hospital in The

Medical Center, in Houston, TX enough times that I had favorite RN's , technicians, doctors and so forth. That said, with my autism and epilepsy, I did not do so well with surprises or changes so I asked the first person who came in the room if I could have a specific EEG technician set up the wires on my head. This female was one I would get into a fun conversation with, so the pain and nuisance in the process of setting up would not be as bad and time would fly by quicker. This made the process easier for me to cooperate and endure.

I consider myself a nerd and I loved when the research team would come daily with this Stereoelectroencephalography (Stereo EEG) equipment for more in depth seizure readings. In this part of my journey I hoped it would not take ten days before having a seizure. Each day was hard to make it through without the research team coming in to ask me different questions that were mostly academic material for brain reading reasons, not education or training.

Chapter 10

On November 24th, my first full day for the EEG test visit, which led to the Stereo EEG test, I was set up by my favorite technician with the EEG equipment. This was followed by different doctors and their student doctors coming in to tell me how much of what medication I was allowed to take, while also telling me that I was not allowed to take any natural supplements, in addition to prescriptions that helped control my seizures. I begged them to please at least let me take my anxiety and antipsychotic medications. I was fine allowing them to do whatever they needed to make me have a certain number of seizures. These seizures were needed to give them the data so that I did not have epilepsy anymore. I did not want to be rude or aggressive with the people trying to help me by missing my mental health medication. Neither did I want to be in flight mode or depression with suicidal thoughts making the team have to send me to the mental hospital while they were trying to deal with my seizures.

After sharing these feelings, the doctors agreed that I could take my mental health medication, but I was not allowed to take anything natural or prescribed to control my epilepsy. The medical team limited supplements and prescriptions they found to be a possibility of reducing my seizure activity. This included any medications that had not yet been proven to work for seizures. One of the medical doctors explained that this medication would impair them from finding the exact focal point of my seizures. The medical team reminded me that the purpose for the Stereo EEG test was to find the exact focal point of my seizures so that I could then see my brain surgeon to find out my options. The brain surgeon let me know the types of brain surgery I could select from to possibly eliminate the seizures.

The medical team reminded me that I would only stay in there for up to the maximum of ten days, depending on how long it took before I had a seizure and the team got their readings to catch all the information they needed. I would have to go through three more surgeries. One was the electrodes implant for the Stereo EEG that I had coming soon, secondly the electrodes removal and the third was for the treatment option I chose. The Stereo

EEG test was similar to the EEG test that most of us with epilepsy get, but with Stereo EEG the electrodes were implanted inside my brain. The reading devices were inside which made them read much deeper areas of my brain where seizures occurred. My case was one where the seizures occurred so deep in the brain that a regular EEG would not show any seizure activity; while doctors watched me and knew for sure I had a seizure. Regular EEG's have external electrodes with a limited reach. These tests had been performed fairly regularly on me since I was first diagnosed at age ten months old; but doctors were never able to read any activity.

By the time these doctors and their student doctors were done giving me their spiel on what to expect and the goals of this stay in the hospital, the anesthesiologist was already injecting me with a large dose of Ativan for sedation in order to get me ready to go for the actual surgery. Internally, I was feeling anxious but as a technician or RN pushed me in my hospital bed into the surgery room, the last thing I remembered was moving to the operating table. Once I was comfortable on the operating table, I was gone like a light.

I was set up with the EEG and about to get my Stereo EEG electrodes in place. The doctors had told me that I needed an IMAP test while the Stereo EEG is still in place. The technicians tried to stimulate different focal points in hopes to induce a seizure. The doctor's team explained, "If we do not get a seizure from you while you are in here, for up to ten days, we will have the IMAP technician come in to see if he

48

can induce a seizure to get us a very good reading of the exact point in your brain where your seizures originate." She later explained, "If we can get this exact reading, we will have the data your brain surgeon needs to determine which type of brain surgery was most likely to relieve you of your seizure activity. Dr. Tandon, your brain surgeon, will send the results and his assessment to Dr. Lhatoo, your epileptologist in order to give his opinion on the best option for you."

Next thing I remembered, I woke up in a room by myself that I later found out was the post-op room where they kept patients to monitor them during recovery from sedation. Family members were not allowed in the room so I started to panic and had episodes related to my high-functioning autism without understanding where I was and

why none of my family members or
favorite hospital employees were there
with me. I was not alone for long
because once I started talking out loud
with my panicked tone, a registered
nurse came in the post-op room to
attend. She told me that they would take
me back to the Epilepsy Monitoring Unit
where I would be back with people I
knew. However, they were required to
keep me there until I woke up in case of
any issues such as me not waking up.
This was a closed monitoring unit that
was protocol in case of any
complications.

    While still in the post-op unit, I
was certain to tell the RN that I was
starving and I wanted to be with my
family again. I could not handle being in
unfamiliar places without my family
there to help out. I told her that part too.
She asked me my name, date of birth,

where I was and other questions to see if I was fully alert. After answering these questions correctly, another person in scrubs came to push me in my hospital bed from the post-op room to the Epilepsy Monitoring Unit. Just knowing that I was on my way back to familiar grounds, my anxiety eased. Of course, once I was back in the room with one of my parents, I was "hangry." That's being so hungry that I appeared angry, to whichever parent was there this time. I remember the first thing she did was hugged and kissed me saying that she was relieved that I made it back alert and alive because neither of them could live without their "Laney."

Next, once we were both comforted by being back together in the same room, I recall being asked by my step-mother, "What did I want to eat?" I remember telling her, "I don't care, as long as it's free of my allergens. I'm just starving and want to eat." Madre, my step-mother, handed me the menu and I quickly scanned it, somehow made a decision in what seemed like a matter of seconds before she called the kitchen to order for me.

    After I ate, I was back to my regular self so I asked Madre for my laptop so I could work on writing and publishing my books. This is when I was editing my book, _Secret to Success: The Evolution of Public Education & the Workforce_ and it was before my business reached a growth point to have an editor who worked under me. I thought the assistant I had before the pandemic, had edited it but, I saw issues that needed to be fixed on the rough draft. I had him back before the pandemic and he made my covers; edited and uploaded my manuscripts;

and uploaded the covers to my publishers for me. I terminated his contract. Prior to the pandemic, I also had a female graphic designer whose contract I had to terminate as well. I was now alone in my writing.

All that time I spent working on my book which was only day one of my "up to ten days" in the hospital. At this point the Stereo EEG electrodes were inside my brain and I was unable to use any kind of seizure control medications or my Vagal Nerve Stimulator device.

Chapter 11

I knew stress usually induced seizures so I worked on my most stressful responsibilities related to my books and administrative tasks for my business because I was determined to survive this economic crisis. As I stayed busy with work, nurses and technicians were coming to check on me and/or give me different directions or updates related to what they read as seizure activities. I told them many times that I experienced dizziness but otherwise, I was just my regular self busy working on stuff related to my job. The nurses asked me questions to test how alert I was and I passed it every time that day.

By the time I was ready to order dinner, the technician that did the first aid care for my head wounds came in to change the wrap. This wrap was what the surgeon had put around my head and chin to protect the actual wounds. The first aid technician shared with me that it was also there to stop the bleeding. The exciting part was when she fully removed the wrap Madre, my step-mother, took a picture so I could see what I looked like without hair, as well as see what those devices that stuck out of my head looked like. I was very curious. From ages 14 to 18 years old I was a model and actress; I posed for the pictures like I would if they were supposed to go in a magazine or something. I loved that part of being in pictures!

After the first aid technician was done rewrapping my head, we ordered

dinner and Madre went to the Starbucks
on the first floor of the hospital and got
me my favorite decaf coffee. Once she
was back with my coffee and I was done
eating dinner, we got to the other
exciting part. I looked at the picture of
myself and saw what I thought was a
beautiful, confident, but bald headed
woman with devices that stuck out of
her head. I loved it!

   The days went by very slowly but
other than the surgery and doctors
telling me what to expect, the plans and
goals, it was pretty much the same thing
everyday. I slept at night, was woke up
around 6:30 a.m. for vital signs, went
back to sleep, and woke up to start my
day between 8 and 9 a.m.. Then I
ordered breakfast. My parent that was
there at the time went downstairs to get
my Starbucks Venti Decaf Americano
and I took the medication that I was still

allowed to take, followed by starting my
work day. I was doing administrative,
digital marketing, and accounting work
that were the most stressful part in my
opinion, with hopes of inducing the
seizure that doctors needed so I could
get out of the hospital. I wanted to return
to spending my days at Starbucks while
tutoring clients and seeing my friends
who were regulars at that particular
location. However, day three came and
went without any luck so I got more
aggressive with trying to induce my
seizures.

Chapter 12

In the morning of day four, I asked Madre to get me a regular coffee since I knew that caffeine increased my seizure activity. I even asked her to get it with Equal sweetener instead of Splenda. I knew that Equal sweetener was another food that caused me to have increased seizure activity. This caused the nurses to rush into my room more often while I continued to do my high stress work responsibilities, eat each meal, drink coffee, drink water and at bedtime, wipe myself with baby wipes. I was not allowed to take a shower as my day to day routine through day seven.

In the early part of day seven, when the RN came to wake me for vital signs around 6:30 a.m., I told him that I had decided I was determined enough to have this seizure. To do that I was going to maximize the brightness of the light on my laptop and on my phone screens that I knew triggered seizures. I told him how I kept the brightness on my devices so low that most people couldn't read or see what I was doing so it helped with privacy, in addition to seizure control on a typical day. He agreed that it could onset seizures and many epileptics are not able to be on electronics for as long as I was on them. My limit was four to five hours a day while he made it seem like that was a lot for someone with epilepsy.

Sure enough, I executed my plan and nurses came rushing into my room even more frequently on days seven through ten. They tested how alert I was each time and I started failing some of the tests. One type of test was for them to say a color when they arrived in my room but I could not remember it many of those times while I was conscious, dizzy and had memory problems.

Chapter 13

Finally, on day ten, two people came in to my room to do the IMAP test while my step-mother was there to comfort me due to my anxiety and autism episodes. The IMAP people were in my room and sending these signals into my brain using a device. They touched my head somewhere on the front left part since doctors already knew that my focal point was somewhere in my front left temporal lobe. The test was to figure out which specific spot or part of the front left temporal lobe had my epilepsy. It would have been a better chance that my surgery options would involve removal of a smaller section or piece of my brain to reduce the risk of being more disabled. The intention was for me to be better and gain more independence with a better quality of life.

The two people sent the signals with the IMAP test in the right spot. I was getting auras after auras, started to climb out of my bed, called Madre, my step-mother, for her to save me until eventually I heard her say, "Sir, she is having a seizure. She always comes to me when she starts having a seizure." He told her, "Quick! Press the blue button to get the nurses in here." I knew then that I was having that seizure I had tried so hard to have for the doctors that I hoped was my last seizure ever. I blacked out and was fully in a seizure like I had known since I was ten months old. It was the same things that I was way too familiar with and beyond exhausted of having to continue this experience.

Next thing I remember, I woke up in the room surrounded by at least ten hospital staff who attended and played different roles to make sure I remained safe, not falling or injuring myself, and woke up to full consciousness. I eventually did, but at some point after waking me someone in the team said that one was a really bad seizure so the doctors rushed in to help me come out of it but they got all the readings they needed. She went on to tell me that they would take me back to the surgery room to get the Stereo EEG electrodes removed from my head. Then I was able to get out of there and go back home to my regular life, work and seeing my friends. I was beyond relieved!

Before I could eat again, the technician was pushing me to the operating room, shortly after, the anesthesiologist put another large amount of Ativan in my I.V. to get me sedated. Like before, I moved myself from my bed to the operation table. I laid down on the operation table with my head between two pieces, turned a bit to adjust until I felt comfortable and then was out like a light.

Like before, I woke up in the post-op room, only this time there was a nurse who checked on me when I woke up. I started a conversation with her about being hungry and wanting to go back to my patient room where I could be back with my step-mother again, but this time it was not as much of a panic or autistic episode. Though I had both emotions to some degree, it was not nearly as bad as before. I had a better understanding of what to expect this time around.

The nurse in the post-op room with me asked if I wanted to "go home." I replied with, "Yes, but I want to go to my room first to order food and eat." After I had something in my stomach and I was with Madre, I would be ready to go home. The nurse replied with, "Okay. Let me get someone to take you back to the Epilepsy Unit first and then start your discharge process."

After I finished eating, the billing manager and some other administrative people came in to confirm insurance information, followed by my signature on financial responsibility forms and other paperwork. This process had been done at the admission stage of my hospitalization but this time was to confirm that everything in the system was accurate.

While administrative staff were there a registered nurse came in with the doctor's discharge paperwork and orders. This all happened on Sunday, December 6. One of those papers was for an appointment with the brain surgeon set for December 11, 2020, which was that upcoming Friday. After all the paperwork and processes were completed, Madre and I packed and I dressed in appropriate clothes for being in public after spending my time in the hospital wearing different pajama outfits.

       I have not really talked about it but that whole stay in the hospital had made me irritable with different health team members, depression, plenty of anxiety and some fight mode. That has been the problem with every hospital stay and appointment for different tests I had to get done that lead up to this point. I had plenty of autistic episodes, too. This whole journey had been emotionally troubling for me. It had also

been hard because of my paranoia of
doctors abusing me, using me just so
they can keep me coming back by
putting me on prescriptions to secure
their own financial well being and so
forth. I have a word processor document
with a total of three pages of diagnoses,
one per line. There were way too many
to remember! With the long list of
disabilities and my seizures that
occurred almost everyday, even with
medication, I was considered
unemployable and approved for
disability income back in March 2020.

Chapter 14

Of course, when we got home, the things I wanted to do was take a shower and spend time with my cat, Precious, my best friend. Next, I wanted to go to bed early so I could snuggle with Precious and be comforted by her soft fur. That was a very precious night and it felt so good to be home with my cat and back on familiar grounds.

I spent Monday, December 7 through Thursday, December 10, 2020, at Starbucks working and spending time each day researching different brain surgeries. I read about the risks, the percentage chances of being seizure free, the daily tasks I would have to incur in the short and long term for managing each operation. For example, one of the operation choices required me to upload data on a daily basis within a specific timeframe or else the data was lost. My research included the bad outcome results and anything else I found to have a well rounded picture of all the realistic possible outcomes. For each option I compared all the outcomes with how likely it would be to be seizure free. By doing this research, I had made my decision to select one of two options among the ones I found on the internet.

I was very anxious! I was stressed and up and down in my mood that whole work week that led up to Friday, December 11, 2020. That day I went to see my brain surgeon for the first time and faced my decision about which type of operation I would get.

Finally the date came and I had taken my Atarax every so many minutes to calm myself of severe anxiety. I was better than I would have been because both of my parents were there, that included my mom who was a registered psych nurse. She knew the questions to be asked that the rest of us didn't know. I, too, was ready to ask a long list of questions I came in with written down in my spiral notebook. There was space between each question for me to have room to have written the answers the nurse or doctor gave to us.

Chapter 15

Like any other doctor's appointment, I was first weighed, the RN took my vital signs and took me to a room, with my parents following behind. She asked me about my reason for being there at the brain surgeon's office. I gave her all the answers I knew but I had to ask my mom, the psych nurse, who answered some questions for me about my reason for being there. I was clueless, in part because of my high-functioning autism. I did not understand things that the rest of the world did, or if I did, my perception was different than what "normal" people perceive in response to the same exact thing.

After the nurse was done with her routine, Jessica, the nurse practitioner, came in and I met her for the first time. She told us that Dr. Tandon was my brain surgeon that had been ordering all these tedious tests and hospitalizations. These had been going on almost every week from February 24, 2020 through December 6, 2020. She told me that he would be in the room soon. He showed us some test results and gave me my surgery options he had found to be the best.

By that point, I was getting both excited and anxious, more than I had already been since I arrived in the waiting room and completed the new patient paperwork for the doctor and billing department. I already took two doses of my Atarax for anxiety so I put on my headphones with my calming music in one ear while I listened and participated in the discussion with the nurse practitioner at the same time.

In the visit with the nurse practitioner I learned a lot about what to expect after brain surgery. She told me about one of the temporary setbacks; six weeks out of work, which scared me because I was, at that time, a one person business. The pandemic caused my business to lose all sales that in turn made me terminate all contracts with all of my contractual working staff. I was afraid of losing the little bit of upward trend in business that I had achieved. My parents reminded me of my disability and supplemental security income, plus their help in paying all my bills to reassure me I would not suffer in any way. It really was a relief and I realized I overreacted.

Eventually, we had very few questions for the neurosurgeon when he came into the room. I panicked! I felt so anxious based on what I already learned and spent the last eleven months with extreme bouts of high anxiety every week. And now I was scared about the risks in my results if I took on this brain surgery that I wanted so badly. This desire I had after July 2020's seizure when I fell down the stairs and broke my left ankle.

Three doctors had said that I was in the one percent that medications did not work for treatment. Dr. Tandon, my brain surgeon, said, "There is a thirty percent chance that you will not be able to talk or read ever again. It's not what I think is likely looking at your PET scan and other tests results, but I am required by law to notify you of any possible risks."

I started to panic again, interrupting to say, "I am not sure I want it this bad." Then Dr. Tandon said, "Here. Let me show you why." Next, he put my PET scan onto the light and said, "Do you see this blue area here?" I said, "Yeah." He went on to say, "This is not normal. This area should not show up on any PET scan. The blue area means there was either too little brain activity to detect it, or that the area was dead and you have zero use for that part of your brain. Fortunately, that blue area is where your seizures are so as far as I can tell that is the part of your brain I want to remove. It does nothing for you besides giving you epilepsy and constant seizures." He paused, looking around the room at the three of us plus his nurse practitioner.

He continued, "Because the area that I want to surgically remove is already dead, the best that I can tell in your case is that I do not expect you to lose anything besides your seizures. In most people, I would see a risk but you are already functioning at home, work, socially and every other aspect of life without this part of your brain. So rest assured I am confident the risk is not going to occur in your case, but for legal reasons I have to make you aware of the possible worst case outcome."

After I heard that, I was still super anxious but it greatly reduced so I went on to my questions for him. "So, what are my options? You make it sound like there is more than one type of brain surgery that I can select from." Dr. Tandon went on to name three different type of brain surgeries. I remember the two that stood out to me the most which were Responsive Neurostimulation (RNS), which was a stimulator that is put into the brain, similar to the Vagal Nerve Stimulator that was put into the

chest area in women to control seizures.
The other surgery he mentioned that I
remembered was a lobectomy where
they actually removed a part of the
brain.

My parents and I asked a few
more questions that only the surgeon
could answer before he said, "I am
going to give you a week to think about
today and get feedback from your
friends and family. I want you to come
see me in a week to let me know what is
your final decision. From there, we will
get you set up with all the other doctors,
a place in the hospital and set an exact
date for the actual surgery."

Chapter 16

We left Dr. Tandon and went with his nurse practitioner to the counter where multiple nurses and other medical people sat. One replied to the nurse practitioner about the date of December 18, 2020, which was exactly one week away from that day of December 11, 2020. They had me come back in exactly a week's time as Dr. Tandon had written. I freaked out again thinking, "Now I have to spend the last birthday that I know I can talk and read at the doctor's office."

After that was set in stone and I was on the long walk between the doctor's office and the parking garage with my parents I told them just what I thought, then added, "What if I can't have a birthday party or this is my last birthday I can read and write? I do not want to mark my birthday as the day I made the worst decision of my life." My parents reminded me of what and why Dr. Tandon had said and the different reasons why any one of the three options that I decided on, would not have a negative outcome.

When we were home, both of my parents agreed that I needed to research all possible outcomes for the options Dr. Tandon gave me. Later, when I gave my dad the full spiel by phone, he said, "I agree that you need to research all your options, but I would like to add to it that you need to make a pro and con list for all of your options using all possible outcomes you can find by spending as much time as possible for the week he gave you. After you find as much information as you can, look to see which options has more pros than cons. Go with the one with the most pros and least cons, even if it has the higher risk while keeping in mind all that your surgeon told you."

For the next week, I spent almost every day at Starbucks with my friends, tutored my few clients and saw all my doctors that I had scheduled for that week. Only this week, I reduced the time I spent on tasks for my books and tutoring company, other than when I was actually with a client. I researched everything I found about those three surgeries. I did exactly what my dad had directed. However, my mental state and health were very erratic. I had a lot more fight modes, flight modes, autistic episodes, epileptic seizures, chronic anxiety attacks and other health episodes, than I had in any other day or week of my life. I saw my psychiatrist and my therapist. Neither one found anything unusual with all my conditions and this major surgery that was approaching. Prior to reaching this point my epileptologist left the clinic. As a result I had to also see my new epileptologist on my birthday to get his opinion on which option he thought was best for me.

December 18, 2020 was the only birthday I did not welcome. Through my extremely bad health from the past week and doing my best to cope, I made it to the big day. By the eighteenth, I had made a decision. I decided which one of the three surgery options I wanted to pick. However, I wanted to hear from both my epileptologist and neurosurgeon which option they found best for me in their professional opinion.

Both providers, that same day at different times, told me, "First, tell me which one you want to choose based on what you already know right now." I told them, and both responded with, "Well, that's good to hear because that's the one I was going to recommend." Only my brain surgeon had asked, "What did your other doctor say? Did you get his opinion when you saw him earlier?" I said, "Yes. He said the same as you and me so all three of us are in agreement." Then Dr. Tandon jumped up and said with excitement, "Sounds like the decision is made. Let's go ahead and schedule the date. Do you prefer any certain date?" I said, "Yes, can we do it early in the week of Christmas so that my mom and Madre will already be off and not have to miss work?" He started to get jumpy and said, "Yes. Absolutely.

Let's go out here and get my team to schedule it,"; which we did.

Dr. Tandon was ready but I was hesitant. While scheduling I asked, "What if I am not ready?" Mom jumped in and said, "We have come all this way to be here over the last eleven months missing a lot of work. We can't miss this much work again so it's now or never." Then I was quick to respond, "Okay. I am ready."

We set the dates for the actual surgery, the pre-op appointment and all other appointments to make sure everyone was scheduled.

Then we left, until our journey is uncovered in _Lobectomy: Best Decision of My Life Volume II_ .